WEIGHT LOSS THAT STICKS

Lifestyle Changes You Need to Make to Lose and Keep the Weight Off

by

PAUL POWELL

Disclaimer Notice:

Please note the information contained within this document is for educational and entertainment purposes only. Every attempt has been made to provide accurate, up to date and reliable complete information. No warranties of any kind are expressed or implied. Readers acknowledge that the author is not engaging in the rendering of legal, financial, medical or professional advice. The content of this book has been derived from various sources. Please consult a licensed professional before attempting any techniques outlined in this book.

By reading this document, the reader agrees that under no circumstances are is the author responsible for any losses, direct or indirect, which are incurred as a result of the use of information contained within this document, including, but not limited to, —errors, omissions, or inaccuracies.

TABLE OF CONTENTS

Introduction 5

Chapter 1 - GETTING STARTED......................................7

Chapter 2 - YOU ARE WHAT YOU EAT 15

Chapter 3 - BREAKING HABITS 21

Chapter 4 - FITNESS YOU CAN FIT IN 27

Chapter 5 - MAKING IT STICK.......................................34

CONCLUSION 37

INTRODUCTION

How many of us have found ourselves sitting in front of the television watching yet another program discussing how to lose weight? Or, standing in the aisle at the store, looking at yet another product that promises a miracle weight loss. How many books have we seen that claim to have the answer or fad diet have we all taken part in hoping that we will be able to lose at least a few pounds?

The truth is, the media has made weight loss seem like a complicated science, but it really is not as hard as they have made it seem. We all know that there is no miracle pill that is going to make us lose weight. We know that fad diets only lead to temporary weight loss, and that most of the time, more weight is gained than lost after a person goes off of the diet. But what we cannot seem to grasp is what changes need to be made in order to lose the weight and keep it off.

We have been told for so long that in order for us to lose weight, we have to restrict our calories and increase our exercise. However, what most people find is that this simply does not work. If it does work, if they do lose weight, when they begin eating normally again, they simply gain all of the weight back.

What are we supposed to do when we feel like we have tried everything and failed? That is exactly why I have created this book. Over the years, I have learned the hard way that there is no quick fix to weight loss, and that there is only one way for you to lose the weight and keep it off for the rest of your life.

That is exactly what I want to share with you in this book. It is sad to say that the generation that are children right now, are not expected to outlive their parents. This is true for the first time ever in history, and there is one thing to blame. That is fat. It is for this reason that I wanted to make sure that everything that you learn in this book is not just for you as an adult but that your children and your grandchildren can use it too. This can be a lifestyle change that not just you make but your entire family! This can change your's as well as your children's future.

CHAPTER 1

GETTING STARTED

I want to jump right into it, and I want to do this by talking about how you can get started. Many people think that when they decide they want to lose weight, they should simply jump right into eating changes and an hour of exercising each day, but that never works. I want to make sure that this time it works.

You will want to begin by setting your goals. How much weight do you want to lose and over what period of time? It is important for you to understand that you should not lose more than 2 pounds per week because if you do, you are only increasing your chances of gaining it back.

How to set your weight loss goals

There are certain steps that you need to take in order to properly set your weight loss goals, and the first is to be specific. You do not just want to tell yourself that you want to lose weight or that you want to eat more vegetables. How much weight do you want to lose and over what time period? Do you want to lose 8 pounds this month, 2 per week? Do you want to lose 100 pounds this year? Make long and short term goals, being very specific about what you want.

If you want to eat more vegetables, what type of vegetables do you want to eat? How many vegetables do you want to eat each day or with each meal? Want to exercise more? How much exercise do you want to get per day? How do you plan on getting that exercise? Hiking? Biking? Aerobics? What time during the day do you want to exercise?

When you create specific goals, you are going to be creating a map which will lead you exactly where you want to go.

The next step is that you need to make sure that your goals are measurable. If you are able to measure your goal, you are going to be able to determine if you are making progress toward it. For example, eating 1500 calories per day is a measurable goal, exercising 30 minutes three times a week is measurable, and losing 30 pounds is measurable.

On the other hand, a goal of exercising more or eating more vegetables is not measurable. Put a number in that goal so that you know if you are doing exactly what you need in order to lose weight.

The next thing that you need to do is to make sure that your goal is actually attainable. So many times, people who are wanting to lose weight or make any change in their lives for that matter, set goals that are so extreme that there is no way for them to reach them. You cannot lose 10 pounds per week. You cannot exercise an hour per day if you have never exercised before. You are not going to be able to cut all of the sugar out of your diet overnight if it has been a part of your diet for a long period of time.

Instead of focusing on huge changes when you are setting your goals, focus on the small things that will add up and make a huge difference, such as riding your stationary bike while watching television in the evening. When you set goals like this, you are going to be able to ensure that you can meet your goals and not feel as if you are giving up all of the things that you enjoy in your life.

You should also ensure that the goals that you set for yourself are goals that you can track. For example, if you want to exercise three times a week for 30 minutes at a time, you can track this. You can track the number of calories that you eat, and so on. Tracking your progress is going to help you stay motivated and help push you closer to reaching your goals.

Goals are not going to be something that you are going to strictly live by. Setbacks are going to happen no matter what while you are working to lose weight, and it is important for you to plan ahead; know how you are going to deal with these setbacks.

One example of a setback might be a large holiday meal. How are you going to handle being able to take part in the meal without completely destroying all of the work you have done? You may plan your calorie intake for the day in advance, know what you are going to be able to eat, and work to make sure that you do not go over your calorie limit.

No matter what type of goals you are setting in your life, even if you are doing nothing more than creating a daily schedule, you have to plan for setbacks because life happens. Things happen in our everyday life that make us stray off of the course we know that we were supposed to take, however, we cannot allow this to derail us. You have to have a plan that will ensure you are able to get right back on track.

As time goes on, you are going to have to reassess the goals that you have set for yourself. If your workout goals are not working in your life, you may need to change them and create new ones. If you are struggling to lose the amount of weight that you wanted to lose in a specific period of time, reassess those goals and determine if you are expecting too much or if the goals were unrealistic.

Creating your weight loss plan

The first thing that you have to look at when you are creating your weight loss plan is why you are overweight. I know, everyone would love it if I could just type out the perfect plan that would fit everyone and no work would need to be done, but that is not how weight loss works.

Most people believe that there is only one reason that people are overweight. However, there are more. One of the reasons that many people are overweight is because they are not eating enough. When you do not eat enough, your body is going to hold on to all of the fat that you do eat. This is commonly known as starvation mode.

In general, people do not realize that not eating enough is going to cause them to be overweight, and they begin restricting their calorie intake even more as they continue to put on the pounds, but quickly find out that this is not helping them lose the extra weight.

We live in a fast-paced world, one where many people find it hard to eat enough food, and while most would believe that this would lead them to being ultra-thin, the fact is that it does not because when they do eat, they are very hungry and eating more than they generally would for a meal. These meals are also often very high in fat and carbohydrates because that is what the person's body is telling them they need.

However, if you force yourself to make the time to eat three meals a day, ensuring that you are eating the recommended calories for your body, what you will find is that the weight begins to fall right off.

I have talked to so many people who tell me that they cannot lose weight unless they restrict their calories so low that they are eating less than a newborn baby. While they might lose a few pounds in the beginning, they can't continue to live under such extreme restrictions and when they begin eating again, the weight quickly piles back on. Most of the time, they gain even more.

The second reason that many people struggle with their weight is simply that they are not getting enough exercise. Again, our lives are very hectic and there is a lot of work that needs to be done each day. While we may be making the time to prepare healthy meals, what we are missing out on is exercise. The reason for this is that most of us live a very sedentary lifestyle. We go to work and sit at a desk in front of a computer, we come home and sit at the dinner table before moving into the living room and sitting in front of the television or our favorite device.

While we may feel that we are completely exhausted and there is nothing more that we could do on any given day, most of the time, the exhaustion is mental exhaustion and not physical. It is because of this lifestyle that many people are struggling with their weight, but there are things that you can do which will help you lose weight. Of course, this means that you are going to have to do some exercise, which can be very simple stretching exercises while you're sitting on the floor enjoying your favorite television show.

Of course, the third reason that people are overweight is because they overeat and do not get enough exercise. However, by following the tips in this book, you will be able to overcome that. Finally, if you find that you are doing everything right but still unable to lose weight, it is important for you to talk to your doctor because there could be an underlying condition, such as a thyroid problem or hormone issue.

Once you have figured out why you are overweight, it is time for you to sit down and start creating a plan. It does not matter if you are trying to eat more or less. You are going to have to focus on your calorie intake, and you are going to have to create an exercise plan.

This means that you need to sit down and create a meal plan that is going to work for you. Whether this is quick foods that you can throw together and eat on the run, or elaborate meals which take extra time to prepare, that is up to you. Once your meal plan is prepared, you are going to want to take a look at your daily schedule and find time each day that will allow you to exercise. This is the beginning of your weight loss plan.

CHAPTER 2

YOU ARE WHAT YOU EAT

We all know that our bodies get the nutrition that they need from the food that we eat and yet, we still put bad fuel into our bodies. Why is this? One of the reasons is because we do not really understand nutrition. The second reason is that many people do not know how to prepare healthy meals, and the third reason is because many people believe that it is impossible to eat healthy while living on a budget.

I want to work a little bit backward here. First, I want to make it very clear that with a little planning, it is very easy for you to eat healthy meals and not bust your budget. Here are a few tips:

1. Buy produce when it is in season, can, dehydrate or freeze it. You will always pay less for produce when it is

in season and storing it will ensure that you have enough to last you the entire year.

2. Take the time to look through your store flyer each week and use it to plan your meals. Ignore all of the processed junk that is on sale and focus on the healthy foods. Stock up on foods when they are at the lowest price, ensuring that you have at least enough to last for around six months or until the next sale happens.

3. Eat lower priced cuts of meat, purchase meat that is on manager special, and reduce the amount of meat that you are eating per meal. Eating too much protein will make you gain weight, and most people are eating double if not more the portion size of meat that they need per meal. For example, in our family, two boneless, skinless chicken breasts will feed 4-5 people. One pound of beef will make two meals. When we do purchase more expensive pieces of meat, we only buy it if it has been marked down, then separate it into several meals.

4. Use beans, brown rice, and other whole grains to make your meals go further and be more filling. We love brown rice and eat it with almost every meal. If I prepare a meal that I do not think will be filling enough, in comes the brown rice. When we began reducing our portions of meat, we replaced that meat with beans and still replace meat completely with beans at times.

5. If you want to make your dollar stretch when eating healthy, you have to plan out your meals. If you do not take the time to plan out your meals, what you are going to find is that you are turning to convenience foods or fast food instead of healthy homemade meals.

6. Broaden your horizons when it comes to what you eat. This was something that took me a long time to learn. Growing up in the Midwest, there were just certain foods that we ate. When I began exploring outside of the box, people thought it was odd, but I found many foods that my family loves, that are inexpensive to make, and that are full of nutrients. Most Mexican foods and Indian foods can be created with cheap ingredients, but they are full of flavor and nutrients.

7. Always make sure that your pantry and fridge is completely organized. This is going to allow you to know exactly what you have and what you need. So many times, people create a grocery list, but instead of checking to see what they already have, they will purchase every ingredient, and this leads to extra money being spent. If you are purchasing items in bulk when they are on sale, you are going to have extra food in the pantry that can be used in multiple meals.

8. Always find a way to use up leftovers. Whether it be taking them for lunch or having them for dinner a few nights later, you never want to throw your leftovers away. It is just like throwing money in the trash. One thing that my family loves is leftovers once a week, buffet style. All of the leftovers are placed on the table and they can choose what they want to eat one day of the week. Of course, I eat some of the leftovers for lunch as well, which means I can stretch my dollar even further.

You can also change the store that you shop at. It is worth driving a few extra miles if you can save a ton of money on your fruits, veggies, and meat. It does take some extra work to eat healthy on a budget, but it is completely worth it.

The second thing I want to talk about is eating healthy meals. One skill that has seemed to disappear over the years is the skill of cooking. However, this is a skill that you have to have in order to prepare healthy meals. You don't have to take a cooking class if you do not want. There are thousands of recipes online, however, I learned to cook by playing with the food and experimenting with different spices.

If you want to cook healthy, flavorful foods, you have to stock up the spice cabinet. Spices are not as expensive as many people think. You do not have to purchase a brand name spice. Check around your local stores. I was lucky enough to find that Save A Lot offers spices for one dollar per jar. Not only are these going to provide you with lots of flavor, but they are going to give you the extra nutrients that your body needs.

In order to learn how to cook healthy foods, it is important that you take it one recipe at a time and don't try recipes that are too complex. Once you get the hang of simple recipes, you can move on to more complex recipes, and who knows, before long, you might be cooking like a chef.

Finally, I want to talk a little about nutrition. Most of us are confused about what we should be eating. Do we follow the food guide pyramid? Should we count our calories? Should we focus on juicing or eating the entire fruit and vegetable? What about all of these whole grains? Are carbs bad or are they good?

Trust me, most of us have been there, including me, and it took a lot of research for me to figure out exactly what I was supposed to be eating and how much of it. However, I want to save you all of that trouble.

It is safe to say that you know what bad foods are and what good foods are, and very important when it comes to nutrition. Foods that are made in a lab by men in lab coats are not going to provide you with any nutrients. Foods that are natural: vegetables, fruits, grains, dairy, and meat are going to provide you with everything that you need.

So, with this being said, if you are starting out with whole foods, natural foods, you are going to be able to skip a lot of trouble and start getting healthy right away. However, many people find that they are addicted to the processed foods they have been eating and struggle to remove them from their diets. We will talk more about how to do this in a later chapter.

The truth is, there really is no reason for you to have any problems getting the nutrients that your body needs if you begin eating more real food and less junk. It is important, however, for you to understand that you can't just add healthy food to your diet. This is only going to increase your calorie intake and make you gain weight. This means that you have to trade the bad foods for good food. For example, instead of having a candy bar as a snack, have a piece of fruit, or instead of eating potato chips, munch on some sliced cucumber instead.

CHAPTER 3

BREAKING HABITS

B reaking bad eating habits is vital if you want to lose weight. Most people do not realize just how bad their eating habits are because they are comparing themselves to those around them, or because they are simply in denial.

The first thing that I suggest that you do in order to break those bad eating habits is to start tracking every single thing that you eat for an entire week, not changing anything at all but being completely honest with yourself. It is also important that you track the number of calories in each food.

One bad habit that people have is eating a lot of junk food. These foods can be sweet or savory. Chocolate or potato chips are great examples. However, when they try to break the habit, they find that it is far too hard because they know those foods are sitting in their kitchen just waiting to be eaten.

How can you break this unhealthy habit? Because so many people rely on their willpower, it may seem as if it is impossible to break this habit, but the truth is that it is simply too tempting for them to not eat the food when they know it is there to eat. The answer... Stop bringing the food into your home. If you know there is a gallon of ice cream in the freezer, chances are, you are going to eat a gallon of ice cream. However, if it is not there, you can't eat it.

So, tip number 1 is to stop buying the foods that you know are unhealthy for you. Of course, it is okay for you to have these as treats on occasion, but they should not be kept in your pantry and never in large numbers.

The second bad habit that many people have when it comes to their eating habits is that they tend to skip breakfast. Breakfast is meant to break the fast that we are on while we are sleeping. It is meant to give us the energy that we need throughout the day, and when we eat breakfast we also boost our metabolism.

Many people think that by skipping breakfast, they are cutting their calories which should lead to weight gain, but the truth is, that is not true. Research actually shows that eating breakfast can help you lose weight and there have been many studies done which show that those who do eat breakfast weigh less than those who do not.

You do not have to eat breakfast as soon as you wake up in the morning, but it is something that you should do every day, and you should eat something that will sustain your body for a few hours until lunchtime. Oats are a great breakfast that is quick, as are eggs, and smoothies, just make sure to add some greens.

The third bad eating habit that I want to talk about does not have anything to do with what you are eating but how you are eating. Spending time eating at the kitchen table seems to have become a thing of the past. Instead, most people find themselves mindlessly eating while they are watching their favorite television show, and if they do eat at the table, chances are that they are distracted by their favorite device.

When you are distracted and eating, it will make it harder for your body to recognize that fact that you are full and it increases the chances of you overeating. Distracted eating also makes it harder for you to remember your meals later in the day, which will often lead to more snacking because you do not feel satisfied with the food that you have eaten. Make mealtime a time when you focus only on the food that you are eating and not on anything else.

Eating convenience foods or junk is bad enough. However, one thing that many people do that causes them to overeat is that they eat straight out of the package. There is no reason for you to sit down with an entire bag of chips or a box of cookies. If these are something that you enjoy, measure out a serving and enjoy it instead of wolfing down the entire package in one sitting.

When you sit down with the entire package, you can quickly become unaware of the amount of food that you are eating, because chances are that you really are not focusing on the food and enjoying it. In order to understand how much you are eating, make sure that you track every morsel. If you measure out one serving and find that you are still wanting more, measure that out as well and track the food as well as the calories. You might be surprised at how much food you are getting through in one day.

Along the same lines as not focusing on what you are eating is the bad habit of eating while you are on the run. Eating in the car, while you are running around the house doing chores, or while you are working at your computer are all habits that should be stopped if you want to learn how to be healthier and be more aware of what you are eating. We are all guilty of it, but it is time for us to make the food that we eat a priority. Sit down and eat your meal before doing anything else. Even if it takes you a few extra minutes each day, you will begin seeing the benefits in no time.

One of the hardest parts of losing weight is breaking our unhealthy eating habits. Once these bad habits are broken, weight loss is easy to obtain. You will be able to maintain a healthy weight as well as a healthy lifestyle by breaking these habits.

However, instead of focusing on breaking habits, most people are much more successful if they focus on creating new habits to replace the bad ones. For example, instead of eating at your desk, make it a habit of eating at the table. Instead of drinking soda, make it a habit to drink water.

Before we move on to the next chapter, I want to talk about the habit of drinking your calories. I am one of those people who used to not eat all day long. Instead, I would fill up on coffee. While coffee does not have calories in it, I was adding cream and sugar to it which meant I was getting 70 percent of my calories from what I was drinking.

By the time dinner came, I was starving, famished, and ended up overeating. I was not getting the nutrients that I needed, and if you are drinking your calories, neither are you. Instead of drinking coffee with cream and sugar, drink it black. Instead of drinking full calorie soda, drink diet, although it is much better for you if you drink water.

Take some time to really keep track of how many of your calories you are drinking each day. You might be surprised at the number of calories that are coming from your drinks.

CHAPTER 4

FITNESS YOU CAN FIT IN

W hy do most people not exercise? Aside from convincing themselves that they are not going to enjoy it or that they are taking part in some form of torture, many people do not exercise because they simply feel that they do not have the time.

The first thing that I want you to do is to take an honest look at your daily schedule. Chances are that you are going to find you have a lot more time than you thought you had, but that you are not using it in a way that benefits you.

If you have never written out a daily schedule before, take the time to do it right now. Write out every single thing that you do each day, from getting up in the morning, to brushing your teeth, to showering at night. Make sure that you allot enough time for each activity. Most of the time, people think they can get about 80 percent more done than they really can. Don't try to pack your schedule, but just be honest about what you have to get done each day. What you are most likely to find is that you have a few blocks, each being a few hours long that you really do not have anything going on. This is where you should think about planning your exercise routine.

Now when you first start out, you don't have to try and push yourself beyond your limits. If you have never exercised before, start with 5 minutes. When 5 minutes becomes easy for you, try for 10 minutes and so on, working up to an hour. If you try to start with an hour, it is going to be too difficult and you are going to give up. The fact is that this is why most people give up when they begin exercising.

Five minutes is all it takes to get started, and no one is going to make me believe that they do not have five minutes that they can devote to fitness each day.

It is also important before we move on to how you can fit fitness into your busy life, that people make time for what they feel is important. If you feel that exercise is important to you and your life than you are going to do whatever it takes to make time for it every day. Even if it means that you get up earlier in the morning or give up a sedentary activity that you enjoy.

The first thing that you need to do is to choose an exercise that you will enjoy. I hate running. The truth is that I hate being outside most of the year where I live because it is either very cold or raining. This means that if I decided running would be my exercise, I would come up with an excuse not to do it almost every day. However, dancing is something that my entire family enjoys and it is something that we can do together every day. I also enjoy riding a bike, but because of the weather, I cannot do that outside, which is why I purchased a stationary bike.

Knowing that I enjoy both of these things, I can tailor my workout routine so that I am able to dance every day and ride my bike while enjoying my favorite television show each evening. If I had chosen an activity that I did not enjoy, I would not be fitting the exercises into my life.

Some people are motivated by competition. They love competing with other people and if that is you, get a group of friends together and start a competition. If you are like me, I do not like competing, especially when it comes to something like my health. I did not choose to be healthy in order to compete with those around me, so instead of competing with others, I compete with myself. Each day, I work hard to make sure I am doing more than the day before, and that is how I have reached my goals.

Put your exercise routine on your schedule and make sure that you actually stick to that schedule. I know how hard it can be to stick to a schedule. When something comes along and distracts you from your schedule, it is very easy to just tell yourself that you don't have the time to do the things on it, such as exercise. However, this is not going to help you lose weight.

Instead, you need to make sure that you are forcing yourself to complete everything on your schedule each day. Personally, when I create my daily schedule, I know that I am not allowed to go to bed until everything is done. Because I live a very busy life, I need to go to bed at a certain time, and if I do not I am the one that suffers. What does this mean? That I make it very clear to myself that if I do not stick to my schedule, no one else is going to suffer but me. After a few nights of not going to bed until late and only getting a few hours of sleep, you can bet that I stopped allowing myself to get distracted and focused on getting things done.

If all else fails, choose to do something instead of nothing. No matter what it is that you are doing, whether it be writing a book or cleaning your house or exercising, doing something is always better than doing nothing. Even if you only exercise for 15 minutes instead of 45, at least you know that you did put some effort into the task, and you did something. On top of this, most of the time what you will find is that once you have gotten started, you will go ahead and complete the task instead of shorting yourself. That is why most of the time when people are struggling with productivity, they are told to just start.

Now let's talk about what you can do in order to find time in your schedule for exercise. The first thing that you need to do is limit your screen time. Whether it is television, computer, or other device time, limit the amount of time that you are in front of a screen. If you can't do that, then as I have mentioned multiple times, exercise while you are in front of the screen. This is a great tip if you do not enjoy exercise as it makes the time pass much more quickly.

Instead of always thinking negatively about exercise, change the way that you think and make those negative thoughts positive ones. Instead of telling yourself that you do not have time to exercise, tell yourself that you do have time to improve your health. Instead of telling yourself that you can't do it, tell yourself that you can do anything you set your mind to.

Work some exercise into your daily routine. One thing that I do every single day is clean my house. While this is a little bit of exercise in itself, it is not enough to make much of a difference. So while I am cleaning, I have my favorite playlist going and often times find myself dancing to the music, completely out of breath, and enjoying the entire process. When the kids are playing outside, I am playing ball with them or working in the yard. I work very hard to make sure that every moment that I am not working, I am being as active as possible, and that I am taking full advantage of every moment of my life, and you should too.

There are also simple things that you can do, such as walking instead of driving. Walk your own dog instead of hiring someone to do it. Mow your own lawn instead of having someone do it for you. When you plan a family outing, make it one that is physical instead of one where you all sit around together.

The most important thing that you can do is to make sure that you are always moving. If you are talking on the phone, pace around the house. Folding the laundry... Get in a few squats, and so on. There are so many ways that you can add exercise into your life if you really look, and the great thing is, you don't have to do all of your exercises at the same time. Scattering your exercise throughout the day is going to give you the same benefit as if you did it all at the same time, and it will help you from getting bored while working out.

CHAPTER 5

MAKING IT STICK

You've done it, you have lost the weight that you set out to lose by following the information that you have learned in this book, but now you have to figure out how to make the weight loss stick. After all, you didn't put in all of that hard work just to regain the weight.

This is exactly why diets don't work. When a person goes on a diet, they change every part of their life for a short period of time in order to lose the extra weight, but what happens when they eventually go off of the diet and begin eating as they did before is that they gain all of the weight back.

It is for this reason that you should not look at what you are doing as a diet but as a lifestyle change. You are not after you lose the weight that you are looking to lose, going to go back to eating the way that you used to or not exercising. Instead, you are going to continue on with this way of living for the rest of your life.

It is only then that you are going to be able to keep all of the weight off. Of course, you may be able to increase your calorie intake once you are done losing weight because you do not want to be underweight, and you may find that you don't have to work out quite as much, but you will still want to exercise and eat healthy to ensure you do not start gaining weight.

Living a healthy lifestyle and losing weight is not something that should be thought of in the short term, but instead, it is something that you should think about as permanent.

You will want to continue to track the number of calories that you are eating each day, as well as the food that you are eating. It is important that you continue taking part in light exercise and that you make sure you are eating breakfast each day. On top of this, it is vital that you continue to weigh yourself on a regular basis so that if you do begin gaining weight, you can make the changes that you need to make to drop the extra pounds and get back on track.

You should never think about the changes that you have been taught about in this book as temporary. This is the beginning of a new life for you, one that allows you to take charge and ensures your health and happiness.

Most importantly, consistency is key. If you are not consistent, if you begin eating junk or putting off exercise, you are going to end up right back where you started if not worse off. No matter what is going on in your life or what you are feeling, make sure that you stick to healthy foods and a healthy exercise routine!

CONCLUSION

The media have led us to believe that the only way for us to lose weight and keep it off is for us to take part in some extreme fad diet or to spend hundreds of dollars on pills that are supposed to make us burn fat, but as most people know, none of this works.

What does work? The techniques that you have learned about in this book are what works when it comes to losing weight and keeping it off. If you want to lose weight, you have to eat healthy foods, exercise and change your bad eating habits. If you want to maintain that weight loss, you have to maintain that lifestyle.

No amount of wishing, praying or hoping is going to make the extra weight go away. There is no diet pill or supplement that is going to replace a healthy diet and exercise. No matter how hard people try to get around it, these are the only ways for you to lose weight and be healthy.

So, the next time that you are tempted to take part in a fad diet, purchase some pill that's promises are too good to be true or restrict your calories to the point of starvation, remember that while some of it may give you some temporary weight loss, none of them are going to give you significant weight loss nor are they going to provide you with long-term weight loss.

The only way and I do mean the only way for you to lose weight and keep it off is for you to follow the information that you have learned in this book. I wish you the best on your weight loss journey and hope that every time you feel like giving up, you can hear my voice in your head telling you that you can do it.

www.ingramcontent.com/pod-product-compliance
Lightning Source LLC
Chambersburg PA
CBHW072025280526
45788CB00007B/2681